It's not!

It's not!

It's not!

It's not!

It's not!

It's not!

It's not!

It's not!

It's not!

It's not!

It's not!

It's not!

It's not!

It's not!

It's not!

It's not!

It's not!

It's not!

It's not!

It's not!

It's not!

It's not!

It's not!

It's not!

It's not!

It's not!

It's not!

It's not!

It's not!

It's not!

It's not!

It's not!

It's not!

It's not!

It's not!

It's not!

It's not!

It's not!

It's not!

It's not!

It's not!

It's not!

It's not!

It's not!

It's not!

It's not!

It's not!

It's not!

It's not!

It's not!

It's not!

It's not!

It's not!

It's not!

It's not!

It's not!

It's not!

It's not!

It's not!

It's not!

It's not!

It's not!

It's not!

It's not!

It's not!

It's not!

It's not!

It's not!

It's not!

It's not!

It's not!

It's not!

It's not!

It's not!

It's not!

It's not!

# It's not!

It's not!

It's not!

It's not!

It's not!

It's not!

It's not!

It's not!

It's not!

It's not!

It's not!

It's not!

It's not!

It's not!

It's not!

It's not!

It's not!

It's not!

It's not!

It's not!

It's not!

It's not!

It's not!

It's not!

It's not!

It's not!

It's not!

It's not!

It's not!

It's not!

It's not!

It's not!

It's not!

It's not!

It's not!

It's not!

It's not!

It's not!

It's not!

It's not!

It's not!

It's not!

It's not!

It's not!

It's not!

It's not!

It's not!

It's not!

It's not!

It's not!

It's not!

It's not!

It's not!

It's not!

It's not!

It's not!

It's not!

It's not!

It's not!

It's not!

It's not!

It's not!

It's not!

It's not!

It's not!

It's not!

It's not!

It's not!

It's not!

It's not!

It's not!

It's not!

It's not!

It's not!

It's not!

It's not!

It's not!

It's not!

It's not!

It's not!

It's not!

It's not!

It's not!

It's not!

It's not!

It's not!

It's not!

It's not!

It's not!

It's not!

It's not!

It's not!

It's not!

It's not!

It's not!

It's not!

It's not!

It's not!

It's not!

It's not!

It's not!

It's not!

It's not!

It's not!

It's not!

It's not!

It's not!

It's not!

It's not!

It's not!

It's not!

It's not!

It's not!

It's not!

It's not!

It's not!